The Blood Thinner Food Guide for AFib

Vitamin K Consistency, Drug–Food Interactions, and a Simple Weekly Eating System

mf

Disclaimer

This guide is provided for informational and educational purposes only and should not be interpreted as medical, nutritional, or professional advice. The author is not a licensed physician, nurse, dietitian, or mental health provider. Reading this guide does not establish a patient–provider relationship of any kind.

Always seek the guidance of a qualified healthcare professional before starting, changing, or discontinuing any supplement, diet, or lifestyle program. If you are pregnant, breastfeeding, managing a chronic medical condition, or taking prescription medications, consult your physician or pharmacist before considering any product mentioned in this guide.

The author and publisher make no representations or warranties regarding accuracy, applicability, fitness, or completeness of the information contained herein. While every effort has been made to ensure scientific accuracy and currency, medical knowledge and research evolve continually. Readers are responsible for verifying information and making decisions in consultation with licensed professionals.

Use of this guide and any information contained within it is at your own risk. The author and publisher disclaim all liability

Table of Contents

Introduction

Navigating daily food choices can feel overwhelming for those taking blood thinners to manage atrial fibrillation (AFib). Many people find it difficult to balance the demands of their anticoagulant therapy with everyday meals, especially when recommendations seem confusing or restrictive. If you're currently prescribed a blood thinner for your AFib, you already know how easy it is to feel unsure about what to eat—and, just as importantly, how much and how often.

A central challenge for blood thinner users with AFib is keeping vitamin K intake steady from week to week. Vitamin K directly affects how well certain anticoagulant medications, especially warfarin, work in your body. Sudden changes whether due to a big spinach salad one day or a skipped serving of greens the next can alter INR (International Normalized Ratio) levels, raising your risk of either blood clots or dangerous bleeding episodes.

But the obstacles don't end there. Many foods, drinks, and supplements can interact subtly or unexpectedly with blood thinners, sometimes reducing their effectiveness or increasing side effect risks. Even seemingly healthy foods or herbal teas can sometimes cause issues.

That's why this Blood Thinner Food Guide for AFib is designed to offer you practical, reliable guidance empowering you to eat confidently while supporting your therapy goals. Through this guide, you'll learn to recognize which food components need special attention, and how to use straightforward meal planning systems for week-to-week stability.

Our focus is on creating a realistic and sustainable approach, so you don't have to fear your favorite ingredients or feel trapped by complicated rules. You'll find evidence-based tools for tracking, shopping, and meal preparation, so you can maintain your lifestyle with less stress and more control over your health outcomes.

This guide keeps a clear focus: it will not address how to adjust medication dosages, manage emergencies, interpret genetic influences, recommend physical activity routines, or explain clinical protocols meant for health professionals. Instead, everything here is tailored specifically for meal planning, food selection, and safe eating practices with blood thinners for AFib.

Here's an overview of what you'll discover as you move through each chapter:

- The essential role of vitamin K in clotting and why consistency is critical when taking blood thinners for AFib.
- How food–drug interactions happen, including mechanisms by which ingredients or beverages can change how your blood thinner works.
- An easy-to-use taxonomy of foods by vitamin K content, so you can quickly spot high, medium, and low sources at a glance.
- Practical pantry management and grocery shopping strategies, ensuring you stay prepared at home and on the go.
- Menu planning frameworks and trackers that help you keep your weekly intake balanced and predictable.
- Tools for monitoring symptoms or dietary shifts that could affect your INR or therapy safety.
- Actionable weekly systems for meal planning and review, giving you confidence and structure for every meal, snack, and supplement you choose.

Ultimately, the Blood Thinner Food Guide for AFib will help you understand which food habits protect your health and which to avoid without sacrificing mealtime enjoyment. Everything has been designed to help you align your eating patterns with your medication requirements, so your nutrition becomes a reliable part of your AFib management plan rather than a source of uncertainty or frustration. Let's begin your journey toward safe, steady, and satisfying meals while supporting your blood thinner therapy every step of the way.

Blood Thinners and AFib—Mechanisms and Food-Related Risks

Successfully managing atrial fibrillation (AFib) with blood thinners requires more than just taking medication on schedule; it demands nutrition choices that support rather than undermine your therapy. Understanding how commonly prescribed blood thinners for AFib interact with foods is essential for keeping your treatment safe and effective.

This chapter breaks down the main categories of blood thinners used for AFib, illustrates the mechanisms by which dietary components influence their performance, equips you to spot warning signs when eating patterns disrupt blood thinning control, and provides practical tools to assess your risk.

AFib-Specific Blood Thinner Categories: Warfarin, DOACs, and Their Dietary Sensitivities

People with AFib are often prescribed one of two main types of oral anticoagulant medications: ***warfarin or the direct oral anticoagulants (DOACs).*** Each class works differently in the body and, most importantly for your day-to-day life, each has unique sensitivities to food, a distinction at the heart of this guide.

Warfarin is a vitamin K antagonist. Its effectiveness is directly influenced by the amount of vitamin K in your diet, since vitamin K enables blood to clot. Too much or too little vitamin K from foods can dramatically affect warfarin's blood-thinning power, making your clotting level (measured as INR) swing unpredictably. Daily consistency in vitamin K intake is crucial for anyone on warfarin.

DOACs, such as apixaban, rivaroxaban, dabigatran, and edoxaban, are not directly tied to vitamin K metabolism. They work by blocking specific clotting factors and are far less sensitive to changes in food-based vitamin K. However, DOACs are still affected by certain foods, supplements, and drug interactions, though these risks are less about vitamin K and more about other metabolic or absorption pathways.

The table below summarizes the key dietary sensitivities of warfarin and DOACs for AFib management:

Table 1: AFib-Specific Blood Thinner Categories

Anticoagulant Type	Main Dietary Sensitivity	Vitamin K Caution	Other Food Interactions
Warfarin	High sensitivity to vitamin K	YES	Cranberry, grapefruit, herbal teas
DOACs	Minimal sensitivity to vit K	NO	Grapefruit, certain supplements

Mechanisms of Anticoagulant Action and Food Component Influences

Understanding why food choices matter starts with the basic action of these medications. Warfarin inhibits an enzyme required to recycle vitamin K, thereby limiting the body's ability to make clotting factors. If you suddenly eat a lot more foods high in vitamin K (like kale, spinach, or broccoli), the medication may lose effectiveness, and your blood may clot too easily. Conversely, if you dramatically reduce vitamin K intake, warfarin may become too potent, raising bleeding risk.

That's why, for most AFib patients on warfarin, the goal is stable, consistent vitamin K from one week to the next, not avoidance.

With DOACs, the main mechanisms involve blocking different factors in the clotting cascade without interfering with vitamin K. Thus, eating leafy greens or other vitamin-K-rich foods doesn’t impact their anticoagulant strength. However, DOACs can interact with foods and supplements that affect how the drug is absorbed, metabolized, or excreted. Grapefruit, for example, can elevate blood levels of certain DOACs, leading to a higher risk of bleeding. Likewise, herbal supplements such as St. John's Wort may reduce DOAC effectiveness.

Common Failure Signals for Poor INR Control Linked to Diet

For those on warfarin, INR (International Normalized Ratio) is a measurement indicating how long it takes your blood to clot. The ideal INR range is specific to each person's treatment plan, but in all cases, it must stay within a safe range to reduce both stroke and bleeding risks. Fluctuating INRs are often a direct reflection of dietary inconsistencies, especially when vitamin K intake varies greatly from day to day or week to week.

Here are the most common warning signs and indicators that your diet may be destabilizing your INR control:

- Unexpected jumps or drops in INR following dietary changes, particularly in green vegetable consumption or multivitamin use.
- Noticeable bruising or bleeding (nosebleeds, gum bleeding, prolonged bleeding from minor cuts) after large shifts in vitamin K intake.

- Difficulty maintaining an INR within your therapeutic range despite medication adjustments.
- INR values that swing sharply after periods of illness, travel, holidays, or social gatherings with unplanned meals.

For those on DOACs, routine INR monitoring is not part of management, so food-related warning signs are subtler. Instead, pay close attention to any new or unusual bleeding, such as tiny red dots under the skin, easy bruising, or prolonged bleeding after minor injuries, soon after a dietary or supplement change. These symptoms may warrant consultation with your care provider, especially if you've begun or stopped using grapefruit products, certain herbal teas, or supplements.

Rule Set Distinguishing Diet Limitations for Warfarin and Non-Warfarin Therapies

Keeping dietary guidelines clear and actionable is a top priority for AFib patients managing blood thinners. Here's a concise rule set to help you immediately distinguish which limitations apply to your therapy:

If You Are Taking Warfarin:

- Keep your vitamin K intake steady to avoid both extremes of "overloading" and sudden reduction.

- Maintain a consistent amount and type of green vegetables week after week.
- Discuss any new supplements with your provider, especially those marketed for heart health, as many contain vitamin K or interact with warfarin.
- Be cautious with cranberry and grapefruit products; these can raise bleeding risk by interfering with warfarin metabolism.
- Avoid large swings in alcohol intake, as alcohol can unpredictably influence INR.

If You Are Taking a DOAC:

- There are no specific restrictions or requirements around vitamin K or green vegetables.
- DOAC absorption and metabolism can be altered by grapefruit, St. John's Wort, and certain other supplements. Always check with your pharmacist before adding anything new.
- DOACs have fewer food restrictions, making them generally more flexible for those concerned about frequent dietary changes, but be mindful of interaction risks from over-the-counter supplements and herbal products.

Blood Thinning Risk Assessment Worksheet: Nutrition-Triggered Disruptions

To help you recognize and minimize disruptions that could impact your therapy, use this simple blood thinning risk assessment worksheet. Periodically filling this out (such as weekly or after a significant change in eating habits) will make it easier to track patterns, identify high-risk behaviors, and make safer food choices.

Risk Assessment Worksheet

1. In the past week, has your intake of green leafy vegetables (spinach, kale, lettuce, collard greens, etc.) changed significantly (more than one extra serving per day or a skipped daily serving)?

   Yes [ ] No [ ]

2. Did you start or stop taking any vitamin, herbal supplement, or over-the-counter product?

   Yes [ ] No [ ]

   If yes, list: _______________

3. Have you consumed any grapefruit or grapefruit juice, cranberry products, or herbal teas not previously cleared by your healthcare provider?

   Yes [ ] No [ ]

If yes, specify: ________

4. Did you experience any unusual bleeding, bruising, or unexplained physical changes (including small red skin spots or heavier periods)?

   Yes [ ] No [ ]

   If yes, note symptom and date: ________

5. Has your alcohol intake changed dramatically this week?

   Yes [ ] No [ ]

6. Have you had an illness, holiday, or trip that caused a major alteration to your typical meal pattern or food sourcing?

   Yes [ ] No [ ]

Interpretation and Action:

- If you checked "Yes" to any of the above, discuss with your healthcare provider whether blood thinner adjustments or additional monitoring are needed.
- Track which specific foods, supplements, or situations most frequently trigger changes and use this knowledge to future-proof your weekly meal planning.
- For warfarin users, any "Yes" response to vitamin K intake, supplement changes, or fruit/tea interactions should trigger a review of INR if possible.

- For DOAC users, focus primarily on supplement or grapefruit-related changes.

By regularly reviewing your responses, you'll identify both the sources of potential disruption and concrete next steps such as resuming your previous eating pattern or quickly notifying your care team when symptoms appear.

AFib blood thinner therapy brings major dietary responsibilities, but the rules become clear when broken down by medication type and mechanism. Warfarin demands vigilant, consistent vitamin K intake and caution around certain interacting foods and supplements. DOACs offer more menu flexibility but still require attention to metabolic food interactions, especially from grapefruit and select herbal supplements. Recognizing failure signals and proactively managing your risk using the worksheet provided protects against complications and sets the stage for stable, safe nutrition planning.

As you move forward in this guide, you'll build on this foundation by learning how to categorize foods by vitamin K content, track your weekly intake, flag risky interactions, and create simple meal planning routines that respect your medication's unique requirements. Empowered with these principles, you can confidently align your food choices with your AFib blood thinner therapy—enjoying both mealtime and the stability your heart needs.

Vitamin K Consistency—Foundation for Stable Anticoagulation

An unwavering foundation of safe anticoagulation for AFib hinges on one deceptively simple nutritional principle: maintain a consistent vitamin K intake. If you take warfarin for atrial fibrillation, the day-to-day reliability of your vitamin K consumption directly protects you against unsafe swings in blood-thinning effect.

This chapter equips you with the mechanistic understanding of how vitamin K interacts with your blood thinner, actionable food selection tools, a weekly consistency tracker, warning sign checklists, and a meal-by-meal self-audit system designed specifically for AFib blood thinner users.

Mechanistic Pathway of Vitamin K and the Clotting Cascade

To appreciate why consistency is crucial, it's important to understand what vitamin K actually does and how it can upend anticoagulation therapy when intake fluctuates.

Vitamin K is an essential nutrient involved in the body's clotting cascade, a series of reactions that allow blood to coagulate after injury. In this process, vitamin K acts as a required cofactor for the production of several key clotting factors (namely, factors II, VII, IX, and X). When vitamin K is present in normal amounts, your body can respond to bleeding by forming a stable clot.

Warfarin, the most commonly used blood thinner for AFib, works by blocking the enzyme that recycles vitamin K. This inhibition reduces your body's supply of usable vitamin K, diminishing its ability to make clotting factors and thereby thinning the blood.

However, if you suddenly increase or decrease your intake of vitamin K-rich foods, it can override the medication's effect: a spike in vitamin K can make blood clot too easily, and a crash can make it dangerously prone to excessive bleeding. That is why, for those on warfarin, staying steady with vitamin K intake is the ultimate goal not avoiding vitamin K entirely, but keeping it level each day and each week.

Vitamin K Sources Categorized: High, Moderate, and Low Levels

Knowing which foods deliver the most (and least) vitamin K is the key to building a safe eating pattern. While vitamin K content varies, the following reference chart segments foods based on their typical serving contribution to daily intake:

High Vitamin K Foods (approximately 100+ micrograms per serving):

- Kale, cooked (½ cup)
- Spinach, raw (1 cup)
- Swiss chard, cooked (½ cup)
- Collard greens, cooked (½ cup)
- Parsley, fresh (¼ cup)
- Broccoli, cooked (½ cup)

Moderate Vitamin K Foods (about 15–50 micrograms per serving):

- Green peas, cooked (½ cup)
- Asparagus, cooked (4 spears)
- Brussels sprouts, cooked (½ cup)
- Avocado (½ medium)

Low Vitamin K Foods (less than 10 micrograms per serving):

- Iceberg lettuce, raw (1 cup)
- Carrots, raw (½ cup)
- Tomatoes, raw (1 medium)
- Potatoes, baked or boiled (1 medium)
- Apples, raw (1 medium)
- Onions, raw (½ cup)
- Most grains, cereals, and animal proteins

It's important to recognize that dark, leafy greens almost always populate the "high" category, while fruits (except for kiwi), root vegetables, and lean proteins typically fall into the "low" group. Processed foods generally contain little vitamin K, but be vigilant about products with added greens powder or "green juice" blends. Use this chart as a visual reference when planning meals and snacks. The aim is to keep the number of high- and moderate-vitamin K servings relatively stable from day to day.

Weekly Vitamin K Intake Tracker for Day-to-Day Regularity

Tracking your weekly vitamin K intake is a powerful tool for cultivating consistent habits and catching accidental dietary swings before they affect your blood thinner. A simple but effective tracker can be set up as a table or checklist. For each day, log every high- and moderate-vitamin K food you consume, with a tally so you (and your clinicians) can spot patterns:

Table 2: Weekly Vitamin K Intake Tracker

Day	High Vit K Servings	Moderate Vit K Servings	Low Vit K Servings	Notable Changes/ Notes
Monday	[ ]	[ ]	[ ]	
Tuesday	[ ]	[ ]	[ ]	
Wednesday	[ ]	[ ]	[ ]	
Thursday	[ ]	[ ]	[ ]	
Friday	[ ]	[ ]	[ ]	
Saturday	[ ]	[ ]	[ ]	
Sunday	[ ]	[ ]	[ ]	

At the end of the week, review your totals. Strive for similar counts day-to-day. If you notice drastic changes (such as a "salad day" after several days without any greens), make a note and consider discussing with your care provider especially if you take warfarin.

Symptoms and Warning Signs of Fluctuating Vitamin K Impact on Blood Thinner Control

For AFib patients on warfarin, irregular vitamin K intake is one of the primary reasons for unstable blood thinning and dangerous swings in INR. Recognizing the body's warning signs early enables prompt action and prevents serious complications.

Symptoms and signs of vitamin K fluctuation impacting your blood thinner include:

- Increased or frequent bruising, even from minor bumps
- Nosebleeds that last longer than usual
- Bleeding gums after brushing or flossing
- Blood in the urine or stool (dark or red discoloration)
- Menstrual periods that are heavier than normal
- Unusual headaches, dizziness, or weakness (may indicate bleeding inside the head, especially if new)
- Small red or purple spots on the skin (petechiae)

If you notice these symptoms, especially after a change in eating patterns (like adding or removing several servings of greens), contact your healthcare provider. Any symptom of excessive bleeding or difficulty clotting is a sign that your INR may be out of the target range and needs immediate attention.

In addition to physical symptoms, abrupt diet shifts even if symptom-free should be flagged for your anticoagulation team. Diet records help them interpret INR changes and prevent potential complications before they happen.

Practical System for Assessing Vitamin K Variation in Meals: The Daily Check Protocol

Keeping vitamin K steady isn't just about knowing the right foods, it's about integrating a reliable, easy-to-use assessment into your daily routine so you catch problems before they cascade. The Daily Vitamin K Check Protocol is a system you can perform in less than two minutes with every meal, especially helpful if your schedule or menus change throughout the week.

Step-by-Step: Daily Vitamin K Check Protocol

1. Before preparing or ordering your meal, identify all leafy greens and high-vitamin K vegetables on your plate.
2. Count the total servings of high and moderate-vitamin K foods.

- High: dark leafy greens, broccoli, parsley, kale, spinach, Swiss chard, collard greens
- Moderate: asparagus, Brussels sprouts, green peas, avocado

3. Compare today's meal tally to yesterday and your usual intake.
    - Is it similar? More? Less?
    - Aim for the same or similar servings as most other days.
4. If you're at a restaurant or eating outside your routine, estimate servings as best as possible and jot them in your tracker or phone. Take a quick note if the meal contained an unusually high or low number of greens.
5. After the meal, review:
    - Did you have a significantly higher or lower intake than normal?
    - Did you skip any usual vitamin K foods?
    - Did you add any new supplements or green powders?
6. Each evening, add up your totals for the day and review your tracker.

    If two or more consecutive days show significant deviation, alert your care provider, especially if on warfarin.

Tips for streamlining:

- Prep weekly salad mixes using the same greens every time to ensure repeatable vitamin K content.
- When dining out, request salad dressings and green toppings on the side so you can control the portion and consistency.
- For special events or holidays, plan ahead by reviewing menus or packing a familiar veggie dish.

Troubleshooting Inconsistencies and Proactive Adjustments

If you struggle with changeable routines (travel, unplanned meals, illness), adopt these safeguards:

- Stock your fridge with both high- and low-vitamin K veggie options. If you missed a serving earlier, you can balance it at the next meal.
- Keep a written or digital log often, a quick snapshot of your plate is enough for a record.
- Use visual reminders (sticky notes, calendar alerts) during periods of transition to reinforce the consistency principle.

If you accidentally make a major shift (such as going several days without green vegetables or suddenly doubling up), do not panic but do let your provider know. Rapid resumption of old patterns is sometimes as destabilizing as the change itself. Instead, return to your usual pattern gradually and communicate with your medical team for any necessary monitoring.

A strong, consistent pattern of vitamin K intake is the cornerstone of stable and safe anticoagulation for AFib patients on warfarin. By understanding the underlying vitamin K–clotting mechanism, clearly identifying high/moderate/low vitamin K foods, using a weekly tracker, monitoring for signs of blood thinner instability, and deploying a daily meal assessment protocol, you transform day-to-day dining into a predictable safeguard for your therapy. Informed dietary steadiness does not mean giving up greens—instead, it empowers you to enjoy them reliably and safely, supporting both heart health and peace of mind throughout your blood thinner journey.

Understanding Drug–Food Interactions with Blood Thinners

Effectively managing atrial fibrillation with blood thinners goes far beyond simply remembering to take your medication. In daily life, the interplay between common foods, drinks, supplements, and your anticoagulant can dramatically shape your safety and the effectiveness of your treatment.

For AFib patients, recognizing and navigating these drug–food interactions is a cornerstone of minimizing risks. This chapter delivers a practical, streamlined approach complete with a comprehensive interaction table, checklists for spotting high-risk foods and supplements, a conflict-flagging workflow, guidance on diagnostic signals, and essential meal timing rules to help you confidently safeguard your anticoagulation therapy.

Comprehensive Interaction Table: Blood Thinners and Hidden Pitfalls

For those prescribed warfarin or direct oral anticoagulants (DOACs), the foods, beverages, and supplements you choose can trigger major differences in how well your medication works. The most well-known issues involve vitamin K, but interactions go much further encompassing unexpected produce, certain juices, herbal remedies, and over-the-counter products.

Below is a focused table summarizing key interaction risks relevant to AFib patients on common blood thinners:

Table 3: Comprehensive Interaction Table

Blood Thinner	Foods/ Drinks/ Supplements	Interaction Description	Clinical Concern
Warfarin	High-vitamin K leafy greens	Counteracts blood-thinning effect	Clotting risk if intake varies
Warfarin	Cranberry (juice/ supplements)	Increases warfarin blood levels, raises INR	Increased bleeding risk
Warfarin	Grapefruit/ grapefruit juice	May alter metabolism of warfarin	Fluctuating INR and bleeding
Warfarin	Green tea	May reduce warfarin efficacy (contains vitamin K)	Clotting risk
Warfarin	Herbal teas (with certain herbs: chamomile, licorice, etc.)	Some herbs increase effects or raise bleeding risk	Excessive bleeding
Warfarin/ DOACs	Alcohol (excessive intake)	Disrupts metabolism, can increase bleeding	Bleeding or unstable control
Warfarin/ DOACs	Turmeric, ginger, garlic	May enhance anticoagulant	Extra bleeding risk

	(high-dose, supplements)	effects (more with warfarin)	
All	OTC pain meds (NSAIDs, aspirin, unless prescribed)	Additive thinning, stomach bleeding	High bleeding risk
All	Fish oil, vitamin E (high doses)	Additional blood-thinning effects	Bleeding risk
DOACs	Grapefruit/ grapefruit juice	Can increase blood levels of some DOACs	Higher bleeding risk
DOACs	St. John's Wort	Reduces effect of DOACs, less protection	Clot/clotting risk
All	Herbal supplements or teas (uncertain composition)	Varied, unpredictable	Unstable control

This table is meant as a practical tool when reviewing foods, drinks, and supplements you might add to your daily or weekly routine. Any new product, especially those labeled as "natural," "heart-healthy," or "immune-boosting" warrants extra caution and, if in doubt, a check-in with your healthcare provider or pharmacist before consumption.

Criteria Checklist: Spotting Problematic Foods and Beverages

Not all food–drug interactions are obvious. Some foods are healthy on their own but become risky when taken with blood thinners. Use the following checklist to quickly evaluate if a food or beverage should raise concern while you manage your anticoagulant therapy:

1. Is the item known to contain high vitamin K (dark leafy greens, green juices, certain green powders)?
2. Does the label mention grapefruit, cranberry, or pomegranate as an ingredient?
3. Is it a herbal tea or supplement containing chamomile, licorice, ginger, garlic, turmeric, ginkgo, or St. John's Wort?
4. Is it an over-the-counter multivitamin, herbal boost, or energy supplement with unknown or variable ingredients?
5. Does the food or beverage promise "detox," "immune support," or enhanced "heart health" through added botanicals or extracts?
6. Is it a new or seasonal product not tried while on blood thinners before?
7. Does it contain alcohol, particularly in higher or unpredictable quantities?
8. Are you considering doubling up on "healthy" supplements (such as fish oil, vitamin E, or omega-3s) in addition to your usual intake?

If you check "yes" to any of these questions, flag the item for a deeper review and consider contacting your healthcare provider for specific guidance. Being selective with herbal teas and "superfood" blends is particularly important for AFib patients on warfarin due to unpredictable interactions that could either block or boost the effects of your drug.

Workflow for Flagging Potential Over-the-Counter and Supplement Conflicts

Blood thinner users often introduce risk by adding over-the-counter (OTC) medications or dietary supplements many of which are not benign. Here is a step-by-step workflow for systematically identifying and managing these hidden threats:

1. Before purchasing or using any OTC drug or supplement, check the active ingredients for interactions with anticoagulants.
2. Consult your pharmacist when in doubt. Ask: "Is this product safe with my prescribed blood thinner for AFib?"
3. Log any new product, including the brand and dose, in a personal medication and supplement tracker.
4. Notify your prescribing provider about any changes to OTC medicines or supplements during appointments or via patient portals.
5. If a product markets strong effects (antioxidant, anti-inflammatory, or circulatory support), consider it a signal to pause and check for interaction.
6. Discontinue any supplement if you experience new bruising, unusual bleeding, or a change in how you feel after a few days of use.
7. Avoid combining multiple supplements targeting similar "benefits" (e.g., fish oil and flaxseed oil for

heart health), as their cumulative effects could increase your bleeding risk.

Remember that supplements and OTC products are less regulated than prescription medications, and ingredient lists may change without obvious notice further increasing risk. Transparency with your healthcare team about every non-prescribed product you use is essential for safe AFib management.

Diagnostic Signals: Recognizing Food–Drug Interactions in Daily Life

Despite best efforts, some interactions may still occur. Early recognition of signals that indicate you may be experiencing a food–drug interaction is vital for intervention:

- Sudden, unexplained increase in bruising or tendency to bleed (such as with teeth brushing or shaving).
- Gum, nose, or gastrointestinal bleeding (red or black stools).
- Unusual headaches, dizziness, or visual changes (could reflect serious internal bleeding).
- Marked or persistent changes in INR test values, even without clear dietary reason.
- Recurrence of AFib symptoms, such as palpitations or fatigue, after trying a new diet product or supplement.

- Noticeable change in energy, balance, or general wellness shortly after adding a new food, drink, or supplement known to interact.

If you observe any of the above, review your recent meals and supplement choices, and share these details with your medical provider as soon as possible. Even blunted or delayed signals can indicate underlying instability in your blood thinning control and should not be ignored.

Rules for Meal Timing and Spacing with Anticoagulant Dosing

When you eat can be nearly as important as what you eat while taking blood thinners for AFib. Proper timing and spacing of medication doses relative to meals can help minimize fluctuations and guard against unintentional interactions.

1. Take warfarin at the same time each day, ideally with a meal that has a similar composition (especially in terms of vitamin K content).
2. Avoid doubling up or skipping meals containing high or moderate vitamin K (such as big salads or green smoothies) around warfarin doses; spread them out evenly throughout the week.
3. With DOACs (such as apixaban, rivaroxaban), follow prescription guidelines. Some must be taken with food to enhance absorption, while others are not

meal-dependent—but consistency in timing improves safety and effectiveness.

4. Separate blood thinner doses by at least two hours from high-dose mineral or multivitamin supplements to reduce absorption or interaction risk, unless otherwise directed.
5. If consuming an unfamiliar beverage (herbal tea, "super juice," etc.), avoid taking your anticoagulant within one hour before or after to minimize unpredictable interactions.
6. Refrain from experimenting with large dietary changes or supplements within a few hours of your anticoagulant dose. If a dosing error or dietary deviation happens, note the time and content, and monitor for unusual symptoms.
7. For those struggling with irregular meal patterns (shift work, travel, fasting), use timed reminders to align anticoagulant dosing as consistently as possible with a predictable meal.

A disciplined approach to timing not just what you eat, but when reducing the odds of sharp peaks or valleys in drug levels and helps stabilize your anticoagulant's effect.

Managing AFib and a blood thinner, especially warfarin, means treating every new food, drink, and supplement as a potential variable. Consistent routines, judicious use of the above checklists and tables, and prompt recognition of warning signals create a bulwark against avoidable complications. By implementing an intentional workflow that evaluates food, beverage, and supplement additions for their potential impact, you become a proactive steward of your own therapy.

The next steps in this guide will build on this foundation, helping you decode vitamin K content in everyday meals, master pantry management, and establish a week-to-week planning system that keeps your blood thinner journey steady, predictable, and safe.

Taxonomy of Vitamin K in Foods—Everyday Reference Guide

For anyone taking warfarin or other blood thinners for atrial fibrillation, understanding how vitamin K weaves through common foods is a non-negotiable skill. Missteps in vitamin K intake, especially abrupt increases or decreases can destabilize your INR, raising the likelihood of clotting or bleeding complications. Yet consistency, not elimination, remains the guiding principle. This chapter provides you with an at-a-glance reference for everyday vitamin K sources, strategies to detect hidden vitamin K, and practical tools for navigating grocery shelves and meal planning with confidence.

Categorized Lists of Leafy Greens, Vegetables, and Fortified Products: Vitamin K Content per Standard Portion

Vitamin K is naturally concentrated in certain leafy greens and vegetables, and is also present in specific fortified foods. Below you'll find a categorized breakdown, organized by average vitamin K content per serving (about ½ cup cooked or 1 cup raw unless noted otherwise). Relying on these categories rather than hunting for perfect milligram counts simplifies day-to-day decision-making and supports consistent intake.

High Vitamin K Foods (approximately >100 mcg per serving):

- Kale (cooked or raw)
- Spinach (cooked or raw)
- Collard greens
- Turnip greens
- Swiss chard
- Mustard greens
- Beet greens
- Parsley
- Broccoli (especially cooked)
- Romaine lettuce (raw)

Moderate Vitamin K Foods (around 20–100 mcg per serving):

- Brussels sprouts
- Cabbage (green)
- Green leaf lettuce
- Endive
- Asparagus (especially cooked)
- Green beans
- Green peas

- Leeks
- Okra

Low Vitamin K Foods (typically <20 mcg per serving):

- Iceberg lettuce
- Red cabbage
- Cauliflower
- Carrots
- Celery
- Cucumbers (without skin)
- Peppers (all colors)
- Tomatoes
- Mushrooms
- Potatoes (white and sweet)
- Zucchini (with or without skin)

Fortified and Processed Foods With Vitamin K:

- Some meal replacement shakes, nutrition bars, and breakfast cereals (look for those listing "phytonadione," "vitamin K1," or "menaquinone," "vitamin K2" in the ingredient panel)
- Plant-based dairy alternatives if advertised as "nutritionally complete" or "fortified"

Remember that serving sizes can make a big difference. A "super-sized" salad with three cups of spinach or kale can quickly triple your vitamin K dose compared to a single cup.

Identification Markers for Hidden Vitamin K in Processed Foods and Green Powders

Not all vitamin K comes from obvious sources. The rise of "green" powders, smoothie boosters, and health bars demands a watchful eye because even foods not traditionally associated with vitamin K may now contain it via concentrated extracts.

Key Warning Signs for Hidden Vitamin K Content:

- Ingredients such as "spinach powder," "kale powder," "alfalfa extract," "barley grass," or "wheatgrass" are high on the ingredient list
- "Green superfood," "detox blend," or "immune greens" labelling
- "Phytonadione" or "menaquinone" (the active forms of vitamin K) are listed
- Claims of "high in antioxidants" or "heart health support" with visible green coloration
- Plant-based protein products with "whole plant blend" or "green veggie base"

Even non-green products such as fiber bars or herbal capsules may list dried greens or green tea extract, potentially contributing hidden vitamin K. Herbal teas containing alfalfa, nettle, or other green botanicals can also provide unexpected amounts—these usually aren't reflected in standard nutrition data, making label reading crucial.

Quick-Access Vitamin K Food Content Wallet Card Template

Consistency becomes easier when you have a portable reminder of "high" versus "low" vitamin K foods. Below is a template for a simple vitamin K wallet card you can personalize and keep handy on grocery runs or when dining out:

FRONT: Vitamin K Quick Reference – AFib & Warfarin

High-Vitamin K (Limit or Keep Steady)

- Kale, spinach, collards, chard
- Broccoli, Brussels sprouts, parsley
- "Greens" powders, green juices

Moderate Vitamin K (Count toward intake)

Green beans, lettuce (not iceberg), peas, cabbage

Low Vitamin K (Flexible choices)

Iceberg lettuce, carrots, peppers, tomatoes, potatoes, berries

BACK: Check labels for:

- "Greens blend," "green superfood," "spinach/kale powder"
- Fortified shakes/cereals with "vitamin K" added

Daily Tip: Keep serving sizes consistent week-to-week. When in doubt, consult your pharmacist or dietitian.

Customize this card to highlight your own dietary patterns and staple foods. Carrying a visual reminder can prevent accidental overconsumption of high-vitamin K items on days you dine away from home or try new products.

Substitution Chart: Swapping High-Vitamin K Items for Lower-Dose Alternatives

Adhering to AFib blood thinner guidelines means enjoying a variety of foods without abrupt swings in vitamin K intake. If a recipe, meal, or dining option features a leafy green or vegetable on the "high" list, use this substitution guide to make adjustments while maintaining taste and nutrition.

High-Vitamin K Food → Lower-Vitamin K Alternative Examples

- ***Spinach (in salads, wraps, or omelets)*** → Iceberg lettuce or romaine hearts (in moderation)
- ***Kale (smoothies, sautés)*** → Bok choy, arugula, or green beans (less dense in vitamin K)
- ***Collard greens (soups, stews)*** → Swiss chard (moderate), or cabbage (lower)
- ***Broccoli (main or side dish)*** → Cauliflower, zucchini, or carrots
- ***Green "superfood" smoothie*** → Banana-berry smoothie with carrots and flaxseed

If your usual dish contains a cooked high-K green, replace at least half with a lower-K alternative and monitor your INR if you plan to make the swap a part of your regular routine. When possible, stick with familiar, moderate-to-low K vegetables for large salads, stir-fries, or soups.

Practical Guide to Reading Nutrition Labels for Vitamin K Content

Although the FDA does not require vitamin K listing on standard nutrition labels, understanding ingredient panels is essential for blood thinner users with AFib. Here's a stepwise workflow to help you decode product labels and spot hidden vitamin K:

1. ***Scan the ingredients list*** for any greens (spinach, kale, collard, chard, parsley) or powdered forms (spinach powder, "supergreens blend").
2. ***Look for the names "phytonadione"*** (vitamin K1) or "menaquinone" (vitamin K2) in both the nutrition facts and the supplement facts, especially on multivitamins, green powders, and fortification statements.
3. ***On processed or fortified foods (plant-based milks, meal bars, shakes), check for "vitamin K"*** among the listed nutrients. If listed, note the amount per serving and match this to your day's other vitamin K sources.
4. ***Be wary of proprietary "greens blends," detox formulas, and "immunity" products***. Unless the exact

vitamin K content is disclosed, treat these as high-K risks.

5. ***Herbal teas and flavored water mixes***: Examine for inclusion of alfalfa, nettle, dandelion, or other green plant names. If uncertain, contact the brand or check third-party databases for approximate vitamin K values.
6. ***For whole produce***: When barcode scanning is available through digital apps, use it to pull up approximate K values, but always cross-check for preparation method and serving size.

Keep in mind that many restaurants and deli-prepared foods may not disclose vitamin K content directly, especially if green ingredients are in sauces, dressings, or hidden layers. When in doubt, ask about ingredient specifics or opt for visible, low-K produce.

Additional Tips for Confident Vitamin K Management in AFib

- Aim for a steady daily intake of vitamin K rather than large swings from day to day.
- When introducing a new food, snack, or supplement, start small and monitor your INR for at least a week before making it a regular feature.
- Beware of foods or beverages advertised as "superfoods," "immune-boosters," or "detoxifying" if they have a vibrant green hue or vegetable powder

blends; these often mean hidden high vitamin K content.

- Avoid relying on generic "healthy" food branding. Instead, reference your wallet card, the substitution chart, and ingredient labels for assurance.

In daily AFib and blood thinner management, decoding the vitamin K content of foods whether fresh, packaged, or "healthified" is a skill that supports not only your INR stability but also your peace of mind. Use the reference charts and checklists from this chapter as your everyday guide to navigating shopping, meal prep, and on-the-go eating. As you build familiarity with these foods and their vitamin K profile, you'll develop a consistent routine that keeps your blood thinner therapy working safely—without sacrificing taste or nutritional well-being.

This mastery over food choices paves the way for the next chapter, where we'll broaden your toolkit to tackle other food elements beyond vitamin K that affect anticoagulation, reinforcing your commitment to safe, predictable, and enjoyable nutrition while managing AFib.

Beyond Vitamin K—Other Food Factors Affecting Blood Thinners

While maintaining steady vitamin K intake is central to safe anticoagulation for atrial fibrillation, there are a host of other foods and dietary habits that can meaningfully alter how blood thinners perform. The challenge with these "beyond vitamin K" food factors is that they're often found in everyday items spices, beverages, fats, and processed foods yet their effects on blood thinner metabolism are less obvious than a bowl of kale. This chapter gives you an actionable guide to recognizing these other components, directly mapping their impact on anticoagulant medications, and building a safer daily eating routine.

Identification Table: Alcohol, High-Dose Garlic, Ginger, and Turmeric

Certain foods and ingredients are well-documented for their capacity to influence the blood's clotting characteristics on top of any vitamin K effects. For those using warfarin or other anticoagulants to manage AFib, keeping tabs on these foods is essential. Each can either potentiate or counteract the therapeutic effect of your medication, thereby raising the risk of either bleeding or clotting events.

Below is a practical reference summarizing key non-vitamin K substances and their interactions with anticoagulant metabolism:

Table 4: Identification Table

Food/Drink	Impact on Anticoagulation	Cautionary Note
Alcohol	Can strongly increase bleeding risk; interferes with liver metabolism of blood thinners	Limit intake to no more than one standard drink per day; avoid binge drinking
High-Dose Garlic	Natural blood-thinning effect, can amplify medication potency	Regular food use is generally safe, but concentrated supplements best avoided
Ginger	May have mild antiplatelet effect, increases bleeding risk with high or supplemental doses	Moderate amounts in cooking are acceptable; avoid excessive intake
Turmeric	Contains curcumin, which may enhance anticoagulant effects	Use as a spice is fine; steer clear of high-dose curcumin supplements

Whenever you hear claims of "natural" blood thinning, remember that additive effects—especially when combined with prescribed anticoagulants—can tip your INR out of range or increase bruising and bleeding. Consuming these ingredients in typical culinary amounts (such as seasoning or flavor) is unlikely to cause significant issues. However, high doses and concentrated extracts present substantial risks, especially if taken daily alongside blood thinners.

Stepwise Approach: Navigating High-Fat Meals and Absorption Changes

Meal composition, particularly fat content, can subtly influence how your body absorbs and processes oral anticoagulants. For instance, warfarin and many direct oral anticoagulants are absorbed in the gut, and their uptake can be modulated by the type and quantity of fat present in your meals.

Here's a simple step-by-step strategy to help you minimize food-fat-related disruptions to your anticoagulant therapy:

1. ***Keep Fat Intake Consistent***: Large variations in daily fat (for example, consecutive days of very rich, greasy meals followed by very low-fat days) can impact how predictably your medication is absorbed. Aim for a balanced fat intake, spreading sources such as olive oil, nuts, seeds, and small servings of cheese or avocado evenly over the week.
2. ***Avoid "Fat Bombs"***: Meals exceptionally high in fat (deep-fried items, creamy sauces, heavy desserts) may slow stomach emptying and alter drug absorption rates. Opt instead for grilled, baked, or steamed preparations, particularly at dinner, to avoid overnight fluctuations.

3. ***Pair Medication with Routine Meals***: Take your blood thinner at the same time each day, with a meal that is typical for you in both fat and general content. This keeps absorption patterns stable, helping maintain your INR or therapeutic range.
4. ***Mark and Track Changes***: If you add or subtract major fatty foods from your diet—say, during holidays or travel note these shifts so you can monitor for medication effect changes.
5. ***Discuss Major Dietary Overhauls with Your Care Team***: If considering substantial dietary changes (for example, adopting a high-fat diet), always consult your healthcare provider or dietitian to anticipate and manage medication adjustments.

Applied consistently, these steps help safeguard against unpredictable spikes or dips in your medication level due to shifting fat intake.

Salicylate and Polyphenol Exposure: Sources and Boundaries

Some plant foods, particularly certain fruits, vegetables, herbs, and spices, contain naturally occurring chemicals called salicylates and polyphenols. Salicylates have a mild blood-thinning effect similar to aspirin, while polyphenols may modestly affect clotting or interact with drug-metabolizing enzymes.

Salicylate Sources to Note:

- Natural in berries (especially strawberries), cherries, oranges, raisins, and prunes
- Found in spices like cinnamon and curry powder
- Present in herbs such as mint, thyme, and oregano

Polyphenol-Rich Foods Include:

- Green and black tea
- Red grapes, pomegranates
- Dark chocolate, cocoa
- Cranberries, blueberries

For most people on blood thinners, regular, balanced consumption of these foods does not require restriction. Problems are more likely when these are consumed in large, concentrated quantities, such as herbal extracts, strong teas brewed very frequently, or dietary supplements containing high doses of isolated plant compounds.

Boundary advice:

- Stick to whole food forms, using modest portions as part of a varied diet.
- Avoid excessive intake of teas known to have high salicylate content if you also take antiplatelet agents or anti-inflammatories, as this combination may accentuate bleeding risk.

- Don’t use herbal or concentrated plant extract supplements unless specifically approved by your healthcare provider.

Checklist: Processed Foods with Preservatives and Additives That Can Interact with Blood Thinners

Many modern processed foods contain a variety of preservatives, stabilizers, and additives. Some of these are known or suspected to interfere with blood thinner effectiveness, typically by altering liver metabolism or gut absorption.

To navigate grocery shelves and meal choices, use this checklist to minimize risk:

1. ***Read labels meticulously for the following red-flag additives***:
    - Sodium benzoate
    - Sulfites or sulfur dioxide
    - BHA (butylated hydroxyanisole) and BHT (butylated hydroxytoluene)
    - Artificial food colors (such as Yellow #5)
    - Monosodium glutamate (MSG)
2. ***Choose minimally processed foods***: Prefer fresh, frozen, or simply prepared items where possible. Canned goods, pre-made meals, and shelf-stable snacks are more likely to harbor additives that could interfere with drug metabolism.

3. ***Limit charred or smoked foods***: Frequently eating smoked meats or heavily charred foods introduces polycyclic aromatic hydrocarbons that may ramp up liver enzymes, potentially lowering anticoagulant effectiveness.
4. ***Watch for "enriched," "fortified," or "supplemented" claims***: Some products may contain added vitamin K, other vitamins, or botanicals that can interact with your medication. Always scan the full ingredient and nutrition panel.
5. ***Spot "natural flavors," "herbal blends," or "botanical extracts"***: These umbrella terms can conceal unknown plant compounds, including hidden vitamin K or salicylates.
6. ***Keep a running list***: Each time you try a new processed product, add it to a notebook. If you notice changes in bruising, bleeding, or INR after eating a product, flag it for your care team's review.

Caffeine and Hydration Consideration Framework

Caffeine, commonly found in coffee, tea, energy drinks, and cola, can influence hydration status and occasionally interacts with cardiovascular medications. While caffeine doesn't directly alter blood thinner effectiveness, it can indirectly influence your heart rhythm and fluid balance, which are crucial for AFib management.

Practical Intake Limits:

- Limit caffeine intake to approximately 200–300 mg per day: equivalent to about 2–3 regular cups of brewed coffee.
- Monitor for increased palpitations or rapid heart rate, especially if you have known caffeine sensitivity. AFib patients may be more susceptible to rhythm irregularities tied to caffeine.
- Avoid high-caffeine energy drinks, particularly those with added herbal stimulants (such as guarana or yerba mate).

Hydration Keys:

- Stay consistently hydrated: Dehydration can increase your risk of developing abnormal heart rhythms and may make it more difficult for your body to process medications effectively.
- Prioritize water, seltzer, or herbal teas without hidden botanicals or excessive sweeteners.
- Balance diuretic drinks (coffee, tea) with equal or greater amounts of water to offset fluid loss.
- For those with additional heart or kidney issues, always follow your physician's individualized fluid recommendations.

Summary Table: Key Non–Vitamin K Food Interactions with Blood Thinners

Table 5: Summary Table

Food/ Drink/ Additive	Risk/Interaction	Safe Intake Recommendation
Alcohol	Potentiates bleeding, affects liver metabolism	≤1 drink/day; avoid binges
High-dose garlic, ginger	May increase bleeding risk	Use in typical culinary amounts only
Turmeric/ spices	Mild additive effects, with excessive use	Regular seasoning okay, no high-dose supplements
High-fat meals	Alters medication absorption and INR stability	Balanced fat intake, routine meal timing
Salicylate/ Polyphenols	Increase in very high doses, esp. supplements	Favor whole foods, modest portions
Processed preservatives	Some (e.g., sulfites) can disrupt metabolism	Choose fresh/minimal processed options
Caffeine	Indirect cardiac/INR effects; dehydration risk	2–3 cups coffee max/day, hydrate well

A comprehensive approach to using this guide means being aware not just of green vegetables or vitamin K-rich ingredients, but the constellation of other dietary factors that influence how your anticoagulant therapy works. When you plan meals, read labels, or consider new foods, measure not just vitamin K but also whether you are introducing significant change in your pattern of alcohol, caffeine, preserved foods, and culinary herbs and spices.

Through this structured approach, you'll build not only safer routines but peace of mind knowing you're minimizing the full spectrum of food–drug risks while enjoying a flavorful, varied diet as part of your AFib blood thinner management plan.

Building an AFib Blood Thinner–Safe Kitchen and Pantry

For individuals managing atrial fibrillation (AFib) with blood thinners, maintaining a well-organized kitchen and pantry transcends mere convenience; it's a fundamental strategy for safeguarding your health. The foods you choose and the way you structure your food environment can dramatically reduce daily dietary risks, help avoid unintentional food–drug interactions, and, most crucially, ensure a consistent intake of vitamin K.

This chapter provides practical tools, detailed checklists, and step-by-step systems to help you transform your kitchen into a place of reliability and safety, supporting your unique needs when it comes to AFib and blood thinner management.

Understanding the Importance of a Blood Thinner–Safe Kitchen

When you're on blood thinners due to AFib, your eating habits must become more intentional. The reason for this is simple: many foods and supplements can interact with your medication, potentially impacting its effectiveness or even posing serious health risks. For example, large fluctuations in vitamin K intake can destabilize your International Normalized Ratio (INR), making it more difficult to manage your anticoagulation therapy.

Meanwhile, hidden sodium, problematic additives, and unapproved supplements might further complicate your heart health and medication effectiveness. Thus, the kitchen becomes your frontline in managing these variables.

This chapter guides you through establishing a kitchen and pantry setup that minimizes surprises and maximizes control over your diet helping you stay both safe and satisfied with your meals. With these strategies, you can confidently navigate shopping, organizing, and preparing food, knowing your environment supports your health and therapy goals.

Ingredient Sorting System: Essentials to Avoid, Swap, and Prioritize

At the core of a blood thinner–safe kitchen is a thoughtful sorting process for ingredients. This isn't just about avoiding high-vitamin K foods; it's about proactively identifying all potential pitfalls and making smart substitutions that support your dietary consistency and heart health.

Essentials to Avoid

1. ***High and Unpredictable Vitamin K Foods***: Foods like kale "health mixes," green juice blends, or large,

sporadic salads can cause sudden spikes in vitamin K intake. If these aren't part of your regular, consistent diet, they can disrupt your INR levels and medication effectiveness.

2. ***Highly Processed Foods***: Items containing artificial colorings, sulfites, benzoates, and other preservatives can interfere with drug metabolism or add unwanted sodium. High sodium intake is linked to increased blood pressure risk, complicating AFib management and affecting INR stability.
3. ***Unapproved Supplements***: Herbal extracts such as high-dose turmeric, garlic pills, and certain "heart health" blends can unpredictably thin or thicken your blood, posing risks if not vetted by your healthcare provider.
4. ***Deli Meats and Ready-to-Eat Items***: These foods often hide significant amounts of sodium, preservatives, and unlisted botanicals, making them a risk for blood thinner users.

Swaps for Safety

1. ***Low or Moderate Vitamin K Vegetables***: Instead of dark leafy greens (unless consumed consistently), opt for vegetables like cauliflower, carrots, mushrooms, or bell peppers. These offer nutritional benefits with less risk of fluctuating vitamin K intake.

2. ***Reduced Sodium Options***: Replace high-sodium canned goods with no-salt-added or fresh/frozen versions. This swap helps manage blood pressure and reduces hidden sodium intake.
3. ***Simple Dressings***: Instead of flavored vinegars or commercial salad dressings—which may contain unexpected herbal additives use olive oil and lemon or homemade vinaigrettes with ingredients you trust.
4. ***Predictable Ingredients***: Build your meals using foods that fit your typical intake patterns for vitamin K. For example, if you regularly eat romaine or iceberg lettuce, continue to do so in consistent amounts.

Ingredients to Prioritize

1. ***Foods That Match Your Routine***: Select vegetables and greens with a predictable vitamin K content that aligns with your established intake. Consistency is key for INR stability.
2. ***Whole Grains, Fruits, and Lean Proteins***: These foods support heart health and are generally neutral regarding blood thinner efficacy. Choose brown rice, oats, whole wheat bread (check for vitamin K fortification), apples, bananas, berries, fish, poultry, eggs, tofu, and legumes.
3. ***Healthy Cooking Oils***: Use olive or canola oil for cooking. These oils have minimal interactions with

anticoagulants and support a Mediterranean-style, heart-healthy diet.

4. ***Low-Sodium and Minimally Processed Products***: Favor products that are low in sodium and free from artificial preservatives and unlisted herbal blends, helping to avoid unexpected INR fluctuations.

By applying this ingredient sorting system, you ensure your kitchen supports a steady, reliable food routine. This reduces the chance of unexpected dietary changes that could destabilize your INR or compromise your medication's effectiveness.

Shopping Checklist Template: Vitamin K, Sodium, and Interaction-Conscious Selections

A focused shopping checklist is your best ally in avoiding problematic foods and reinforcing healthy choices. Use the following template to plan your grocery runs and protect yourself against the most common blood thinner pitfalls:

1. ***Fresh or Frozen Low–Vitamin K Vegetables***: Cauliflower, zucchini, eggplant, green beans, peppers.
2. ***Moderate–Vitamin K Choices***: Broccoli, brussels sprouts (if eaten regularly and in consistent, set amounts).
3. ***Fruits***: Apples, bananas, peaches, berries all typically low in vitamin K and safe if eaten consistently.

4. ***Proteins***: Skinless poultry, fish, eggs, tofu, legumes. Prepare without high-sodium sauces or cured meats.
5. ***Dairy***: Low-fat milk, yogurt, small quantities of cheese. Avoid processed cheese with hidden additives.
6. ***Whole Grains***: Brown rice, oats, whole wheat bread (double-check labels for vitamin K enrichment).
7. ***Heart-Healthy Oils***: Olive, canola, avocado oil.
8. ***Unsalted Nuts and Seeds***: Choose plain varieties without added salt or flavoring.
9. ***No-Salt–Added Canned Goods***: Tomatoes, beans, or vegetables.
10. ***Condiments***: Plain mustard, vinegar, lemon or lime juice.

Foods to Avoid:

- Green "superfood" powders
- Unapproved supplements
- Herbal teas of unknown vitamin K content
- Canned soups, pickled/deli items high in sodium or preservatives
- Products making "heart health boost" claims without detailed ingredient information

Tip: Bring this list with you on every shopping trip, and take a moment to mark packages or produce with a note about their vitamin K and sodium content. This makes meal planning and preparation at home smoother and safer.

Storage Guide for Herbs, Greens, and Supplements

One of the most common sources of unplanned dietary changes is the variable supply and freshness of perishable foods especially greens and herbs that contain significant vitamin K. A deliberate storage system can help reduce waste, extend shelf life, and keep your intake consistent.

Leafy Greens:

- Wash and thoroughly dry greens before storage.
- Store in clear, sealed containers with a dry paper towel to absorb moisture.
- Divide into daily-use portions to preserve freshness and reinforce regular consumption patterns.

Herbs:

- Store fresh herbs upright in a small glass of water in the refrigerator, loosely covered with a plastic bag.
- For dried herbs and spices, keep in airtight containers away from light and heat to prevent potency loss or fluctuations.

Supplements:

- Only store supplements prescribed or approved by your healthcare team in a designated area separate from regular pantry items.

- Keep a written list detailing supplement start dates and daily doses. This helps you quickly spot any changes that might affect your INR stability.

Back-Stock Items:

- Avoid keeping surplus vitamin K–rich greens or unapproved supplements that might tempt you to increase consumption impulsively.
- Purchase only what you expect to use in a week, reinforcing dietary consistency and reducing waste.

Label Review Checklist for Ready-Made and Deli Products

Many ready-made, deli, and packaged foods are sources of hidden vitamin K, sodium, botanicals, and preservatives. A blood thinner–safe kitchen relies on methodical label review before any new item enters your home:

1. Scan for all forms of vitamin K on ingredient panels ("phylloquinone," "menadione," "K1/K2").
2. Check sodium levels, aiming for products under 140 mg sodium per serving. Some individuals may need to follow stricter limits as advised by their healthcare provider.
3. Identify preservatives: Sulfites, sodium benzoate, nitrates, and BHA/BHT are best avoided as they can alter how your body processes medications.

4. Watch for "herbal blends," "supergreens," or "natural flavors"—these phrases often signal unlisted botanicals or vitamin K-containing concentrates.
5. If nutrition data is missing or unclear (such as with deli counter salads or prepared foods), request a detailed ingredient list from staff or skip the item in favor of a known-safe choice.
6. Prioritize brands or products carrying heart-health or AFib safety certifications. Keep a running "green" or "yellow" list of frequently purchased safe products for quick reference during future shopping trips.

Monthly Pantry Audit Tool: Expired, Contaminated, or Interaction-Prone Items

A regular, scheduled pantry audit is essential for ensuring that expired, risky, or previously overlooked sources of problematic ingredients don't find their way into your meals. A thorough monthly check-up prevents accidental exposure, particularly with processed or infrequently used foods. Use the following audit tool:

1. ***Check Expiry Dates***: Remove any foods, supplements, or mixes past their "best by" or expiration dates.
2. ***Inspect for Physical Contamination***: Discard items with signs of spoilage, off-odors, moisture infiltration, or infestation. These not only pose safety risks but may

also prompt you to opt for quick, less-controlled food sources.

3. ***Vitamin K Audit***: Separate high-vitamin K foods and check if their consumption matches your regular weekly allowance. Remove or portion as needed to prevent fluctuations in intake.
4. ***Additive and Preservative Review***: Remove food products containing high levels of artificial preservatives or ingredient lists filled with unrecognized or unvetted flavors, colors, or "proprietary blends."
5. ***Supplement Check***: Review all vitamin, mineral, and herbal supplement labels. Remove anything not explicitly approved by your healthcare team, or leftover supplements kept "just in case."
6. ***Track Interaction-Prone Foods***: Maintain a list of products that have caused INR or symptom fluctuations in the past weeks. Rotate these out or place them in a "hold" bin for team review if you're uncertain about their safety.

Place this checklist in your pantry or on a kitchen bulletin board as a ready reference. Schedule your audit for the same week each month to establish a consistent routine and ensure nothing slips through the cracks.

Additional Tips for a Blood Thinner–Safe Kitchen

- ***Keep a dedicated logbook or meal diary*** where you note your daily intake of vitamin K–rich foods, sodium, and any new supplements. This can help you and your healthcare team spot patterns or potential issues early.
- ***Educate other household members or caregivers*** about your dietary restrictions and the importance of consistency, so they can support your efforts and help prevent accidental exposure to risky foods.
- ***Consider color-coding storage containers or shelves*** (for example, red for high-vitamin K foods, yellow for moderate, and green for low) to make it easier to track what you have on hand and prevent mix-ups during meal preparation.
- ***Prepare batch meals or snacks using safe ingredients and freeze in labeled***, single-serving portions. This not only saves time but also ensures you always have a reliable, safe option available, reducing the temptation to resort to less-controlled foods.
- ***If dining out or eating at social gatherings***, bring a list of safe foods or communicate your needs to hosts in advance. When in doubt, eat before you go or bring your own meal to maintain consistency.

Maintaining a blood thinner safe kitchen and pantry is not about rigid restriction, it's about establishing supportive routines and making informed selections that align with your therapy goals. With smart ingredient sorting, focused shopping, mindful storage, diligent label reading, and regular audits, you'll create a kitchen environment designed to boost your consistency, reduce risk, and empower your control over both AFib and your overall health.

Using these targeted systems, your kitchen becomes a cornerstone of safe, enjoyable, and stable nutrition throughout your blood thinner journey. You gain peace of mind, knowing that you are taking proactive steps every day to manage your condition and support your well-being one meal, one shopping trip, and one organized pantry shelf at a time.

Step-by-Step Weekly Meal Planning System for Blood Thinner Users

Effectively managing nutrition when living with AFib and using blood thinners requires more than simply knowing which foods to prioritize or avoid. It's about building sustainable, repeatable systems that navigate both medication safety and enjoyable eating.

A robust weekly meal-planning process not only maintains vitamin K consistency but also flags food–drug interactions, keeps portion sizes on track, and offers a structure for self-monitoring progress and pitfalls. This chapter outlines a practical, step-by-step meal planning system tailored for people taking anticoagulants for AFib, driving steady daily routines, greater food confidence, and reliable therapy outcomes.

Seven-Day Meal-Planning Worksheet: Vitamin K and Interaction Alerts

Begin with a clear, user-friendly worksheet designed specifically for a full week of blood thinner–safe eating. The worksheet's core function is to organize each day's meals and snacks, highlight vitamin K content per meal, and flag any ingredients that may pose interaction risks with your anticoagulant regimen.

The typical layout includes daily columns divided into breakfast, lunch, dinner, and snacks. For each meal:

- List every main ingredient and commonly used condiments.
- Beside each item, note its approximate vitamin K content using a simple scale (low, moderate, high). For example, "spinach (high K), grilled chicken (low K), brown rice (low K)".
- Flag any item known to interact with anticoagulants, such as grapefruit, cranberry products, herbal teas with unknown contents, or foods with high levels of garlic, ginger, or turmeric.
- Designate a "consistency check" box for each meal, asking: Am I repeating the usual choices or introducing something new? This simple check helps keep routines stable.

The worksheet should also feature a daily total of the accumulation of vitamin K in all meals and snacks for each day helping you see at a glance whether intake is even across the week. This helps prevent sudden increases or drops, which could destabilize your INR and overall blood thinner management.

Iterative Menu Template for Weekly "Safe Meal" Cycles

Once the worksheet is in use, create a repeatable, iterative menu template—a master list of "safe meals" you rotate through with only slight variations. Pick recipes and food combinations that meet both your taste preferences and vitamin K consistency goals. The advantage of an iterative menu is simple: reducing decision fatigue, minimizing the risk of accidental dietary changes, and allowing swift troubleshooting if your INR becomes unstable.

Follow these steps to build your menu cycle:

1. ***Identify five to eight meals (breakfasts, lunches, dinners)*** that you enjoy, know to be safe, and which use ingredients with predictable vitamin K content.
2. ***Plan for two or three consistent snacks each week***, such as a small apple, a plain yogurt, or carrot sticks each marked for known vitamin K status.
3. ***Rotate your chosen meals*** throughout the seven days in different arrangements, using only minor swaps

(e.g., substituting chicken for fish, or rotating among "low K" vegetables).

4. ***When introducing a new recipe, test it on a single day***, then monitor your INR response before making it a regular feature.

The iterative template transforms complicated meal variety into an easy-to-follow rhythm, supporting stable nutrition patterns week after week. Over time, you'll gain the confidence that comes from a known, tested food cycle, reducing INR surprises and food anxiety.

Example Grocery List: Cross-Referencing Vitamin K Content

Successful blood thinner meal planning goes hand in hand with grocery shopping that is both efficient and safe. Construct a master grocery list each week that cross-references vitamin K levels for every major ingredient tied to your planned menus.

Structure your list first by grouping foods by vitamin K category:

- ***Low–Vitamin K*** (safe for most daily use): apples, bananas, rice, pasta, potatoes, cauliflower, bell pepper, mushrooms, eggs, chicken breast.

- ***Moderate–Vitamin K*** (include in precise, pre-planned amounts): broccoli, brussels sprouts, green beans, peas.
- ***High–Vitamin K*** (only if your intake is consistently high and approved by your care provider): spinach, kale, collard greens, parsley.

For each food on your menu, jot a simple ***"L", "M", or "H"*** next to its itemization ***(for low, moderate, or high vitamin K).*** Include separate symbols for foods or ingredients that are interaction risks—such as ***"G" for grapefruit*** or ***"H" for herbal teas.***

An example of a cross-referenced grocery list based on a stable weekly plan:

- Chicken breast (L)
- Brown rice (L)
- Cauliflower (L)
- Green beans (M)
- Broccoli (M)
- Romaine lettuce (M)
- Greek yogurt (L)
- Eggs (L)
- Whole wheat bread (L)
- Apples (L)
- Bananas (L)
- Carrots (L)
- Olive oil (L)

- Grapefruit (*G)
- Mixed salad greens (*H if contains spinach/kale)
- Lemon juice (L)
- Unsalted nuts (L)
- Tofu (L)
- Fresh parsley (*H—use only if intake is stable and approved)

When shopping, use this coded system to quickly remind yourself to keep vitamin K intake within planned ranges, only purchase moderate- or high-Vitamin K foods in amounts you'll actually use, and avoid impulse buys that might disrupt your established cycle. Moreover, by labeling potential interaction foods right on your list, you give yourself a quick warning to double-check recipes and avoid accidental exposures.

Portion Control Signals: Keeping Intake Steady and Stable

Beyond food selection, portion control is crucial for maintaining day-to-day stability in vitamin K intake and overall dietary safety. Even low–vitamin K foods, if eaten in wildly varying amounts, can introduce unplanned changes. Establish visual or quantitative cues for serving sizes:

- Use measuring cups or a kitchen scale—e.g., 1 cup chopped broccoli for moderate vitamin K, 3 ounces of cooked chicken for protein portions.

- For produce, use familiar markers: a medium apple, half a plate of rice, or a "thumb-size" serving of nuts.
- Distribute leafy greens or high-vitamin K vegetables into pre-portioned containers or bags (for example, seven equal bags for seven salads).
- Mark serving sizes on your meal-planning worksheet, so that as the week unfolds, you can quickly check that each day's intake closely matches your established pattern.
- Commit to eating meals and snacks at regular times whenever possible; this helps your body's drug metabolism remain predictable and can prevent both unplanned hunger and accidental extra portions.

Be especially vigilant with foods that have even moderate vitamin K content. If you adjust a portion—say, more broccoli at dinner, note the change immediately and watch your INR more closely in the following days. Over time, these habits help to eliminate dietary "noise" that confuses symptom management and complicates medication effectiveness.

Weekly Review Journal: Tracking Meals, Snacks, and Supplements

To round out your meal-planning system, set aside a few minutes each week for a structured review of everything you've consumed, meals, snacks, and especially supplements.

A weekly review journal is your accountability tool: it helps you spot creeping changes, overlooked exposures, or places where your routine is slipping out of sync with your care plan.

Your weekly review journal should include:

- ***A written log of what you ate each day*** (can copy from your meal planner), with vitamin K and interaction flags clearly noted.
- ***A supplement tracker did you take anything different or new*** (multivitamins, herbal pills, prescribed or otherwise)?
- ***Symptom notes***: Any unusual bruising, bleeding, palpitations, or new symptoms that correlate with missed meals, food changes, or skipped snacks?
- ***Reflections on routine***: Did you eat out unexpectedly, swap a homemade meal for a packaged option, or indulge in a food that is usually avoided?
- ***Plans for improvement***: Based on the week's patterns, what will you keep the same, and where will you nudge your routine for safety or simplicity?

This process encourages active engagement with your nutrition, turning blood thinner therapy into a manageable component of daily life and enabling rapid response to emerging issues. Bring your journal or a summary to appointments with your care provider to ensure you have a complete, honest picture for shared decision-making.

Over time, these planning, shopping, portion, and review tools become habits that powerfully support safe, stable nutrition for anyone managing AFib anticoagulation. With a standardized worksheet, a reusable weekly menu cycle, careful shopping supported by vitamin K cross-references, steady portion signals, and a thoughtful journal, you take control of your dietary routine.

Embrace small, incremental changes and steadiness is the key. The result isn't dull repetition, but reliable safety and the ability to enjoy food without the daily anxiety of unknown risk. Each system outlined above has been built with evidence and dietitian guidance for blood thinner users in AFib, supporting the stability and effectiveness of your overall therapy and your ongoing quality of life.

Monitoring, Adjustment, and Communication with Care Providers

Living with atrial fibrillation (AFib) and managing blood thinner therapy is an ongoing journey, not a one-time event. Safe and consistent dietary patterns are only as reliable as your ability to monitor, review, and adjust them in real time. The tools and techniques in this chapter are designed to help you track critical wellness signals, roll out new nutrition changes safely, and maintain open, effective communication with your healthcare team ensuring your blood thinner food plan works for you, not against you.

Self-Monitoring Guide for Tracking INR and Symptom Logs in Relation to Meals

Regular self-monitoring is the foundation for safe blood thinner management in AFib. Your International Normalized Ratio (INR) reflects how effectively your blood thinners are working to prevent harmful clots especially critical for those on warfarin, which is highly sensitive to dietary vitamin K.

While people on direct oral anticoagulants (DOACs) don't require regular INR checks, food and symptom logs still provide valuable insights whenever medications or dietary routines change.

Here's how to structure your self-monitoring for best results:

- Log each meal and snack, including approximate vitamin K content based on your prior meal-planning system. Mark high, moderate, or low vitamin K next to each item.
- Record the time of each meal, particularly if you are taking warfarin or have meals closely tied to your medication schedule.
- After you collect your INR reading (at home or through your provider), jot it down next to each day's food log. Over time, you'll be able to spot patterns: was your INR stable when vitamin K intake was even? Did a spike or drop in INR follow a dietary change?
- Maintain a log of symptoms such as unusual bruising, bleeding, palpitations, extreme fatigue, or new shortness of breath. Note if symptoms coincide with meal changes, missed doses, or new supplements.
- If you try new foods or supplements, flag these entries, as they may help explain future INR fluctuations or unexpected symptoms.

Tracking both numbers (like your INR) and experiences (like symptoms) helps you detect subtle signals your body and medication are sending alerts that often precede bigger health events. Thorough logs also assist your care team in understanding the broader picture and tailoring advice for your situation.

Timeline for Safe Dietary Change Roll-Out to Prevent Abrupt INR Fluctuations

Sudden shifts in diet such as increasing leafy green vegetable consumption or adding a new supplement can destabilize your INR, leading to elevated bleeding or clotting risks. The safest way to introduce dietary changes is through a deliberate, phased timeline. This approach minimizes risk and allows you and your care provider to monitor for untoward trends.

The recommended approach:

1. Make only one dietary adjustment at a time. If you want to start eating a new vegetable or increase your servings of a certain food, do so in controlled portions.
2. Wait at least one to two weeks before evaluating the impact of this change on your INR and symptom profile.
3. During this period, keep food, INR, and symptom logs up to date and bring any abnormal readings or symptoms such as unexplained bruising or fatigue to your provider's attention as soon as possible.

4. Avoid making additional major changes to your diet, supplement regimen, or eating schedule until you've observed a stable response to the initial adjustment.
5. If you wish to introduce more complex changes (like adopting a new meal pattern or incorporating several new foods), build them sequentially, never all at once.

This cautious, incremental approach allows you and your provider to quickly recognize and reverse any problematic changes before they can cause harm.

Communication Checklist for Sharing Food Logs and Concerns with Healthcare Professionals

Proactive communication is essential for effective anticoagulation management—especially when diet, medications, and symptoms all interact. Use a structured communication checklist during appointments and whenever you reach out to your healthcare provider. This ensures no important detail is lost or forgotten.

Key items for your checklist:

- Bring your most recent food and snack logs, organized by day, with vitamin K content and interaction risk flags visible.
- Provide an updated log of your INR readings (if applicable), aligned with your food log dates.

- Note any new or discontinued supplements, including herbal products, vitamins, or over-the-counter remedies.
- Document key symptoms, especially new bruising, bleeding, irregular heart beats, overwhelming fatigue, or shortness of breath along with the dates they occurred.
- Identify any upcoming changes you anticipate, such as travel, planned changes to meal routines, or medication adjustments.
- List specific concerns or questions: Are you unsure about the safety of certain foods? Did you notice an unexpected INR reading after eating out?
- Note any episodes when you missed a dose of medication, skipped meals, or consumed unplanned foods or drinks that interact with your therapy.

Following this checklist equips your care team with the context they need to give safe, accurate advice and tailor your care plan to your day-to-day life. Good documentation supports both your own review and more informed provider input.

Adjustment Signals for Modifying Meal Plans Based on INR Results or New Medications

Adapting your meal plan quickly and safely in response to changing INR levels or new medications is an essential skill for anyone with AFib on blood thinners. Watch for clear signals that warrant proactive meal plan adjustments, then act systematically to protect your therapy's effectiveness.

Adjustment signals include:

- A sudden, unexplained change in your INR that follows a new food introduced, a significant deviation in vitamin K intake, or a medication adjustment.
- New symptoms, such as unexplained bruising, prolonged nosebleeds, blood in stool or urine, or fatigue beyond your baseline especially if a dietary change preceded these events.
- A care provider's recommendation to boost or reduce vitamin K intake due to long-term INR trends or medication changes.
- The addition of medications (including antibiotics, anti-seizure drugs, or certain cholesterol medications) known to interact with anticoagulants requires you to monitor your diet more closely.
- Major changes in your eating routine such as fasting, skipping meals, binge eating, or periods of illness that disrupt regular intake patterns.

How to respond:

- Pause any new dietary introductions if your INR becomes unstable or if you experience concerning symptoms.
- Temporarily revert to your prior, stable meal pattern, as documented in your meal logs, until you regain INR stability.
- Consult your care provider promptly whenever you notice a persistent change in INR or symptoms that do not resolve with return to your previous routine.
- For planned medication additions, proactively discuss in advance how these might affect food interactions and whether you should further adjust vitamin K intake.

Practicing flexibility with routine adjustments and knowing when to seek medical guidance empowers you to keep your blood thinner management on track, even as your health needs change.

Emergency Contact and Action Card Template for Nutrition-Triggered Issues

Rapid recognition and response to nutrition-triggered complications with your blood thinners can be lifesaving. A wallet-sized emergency contact and action card ensures that you, your loved ones, and any first responders have instant access to vital information if you experience a sudden INR-related episode or food–drug reaction.

Your customizable action card should include:

1. Your full name, date of birth, and a "Medical Alert – Blood Thinner for AFib" statement.
2. Current anticoagulant medication (name and dose), with known food sensitivities or notable interactions (e.g., warfarin—monitor vitamin K, avoid large vitamin K fluctuations).
3. Key emergency contacts: your primary care provider, cardiologist, and at least one family member.
4. Allergies (if applicable).
5. Space to write your most recent INR range (if on warfarin) or any special notes regarding dietary triggers (such as "avoid grapefruit and cranberry").
6. Itemized emergency actions:
    - If abnormal bleeding, black stools, or severe bruising develop: stop all food and drug intake, call emergency services, and present this card.
    - If severe palpitations or fainting occur, call 911 immediately.
    - Note to medical personnel: Patient is on blood thinner for AFib; recent dietary changes or supplement exposures may explain abnormal bleeding or INR instability.

Carry this card with you at all times. Review and update it after medication or major diet changes, or with each new lab or clinic visit. Sharing copies with family or close contacts ensures help will always have access to critical care information when seconds count.

Monitoring, adjustment, and communication are the "active ingredients" in a safe, sustainable blood thinner food system for AFib. Consistent log-keeping, careful pace with dietary changes, regular communication using structured checklists, and readiness with an actionable emergency plan are the pillars of true confidence. These habits ensure you not only respond to problems, but also prevent many from occurring, empowering you to continue enjoying food, supporting your therapy, and maintaining your well-being over the long term.

Handling Eating Out, Travel, and Holiday Meals on Blood Thinners

Navigating food choices outside your home can be particularly challenging when managing atrial fibrillation (AFib) with blood thinners. The unpredictability of restaurant recipes, travel disruptions, and festive meals often introduce major swings in vitamin K intake or problematic food–drug interactions. Mastering a few proactive strategies will help you maintain dietary consistency, keep your anticoagulant therapy effective, and enjoy social experiences with less worry.

Eating-Out Ordering Guide with Vitamin K Scoring Cues for Menu Items

Dining out while on blood thinners, especially warfarin, calls for careful scrutiny of menu items due to the variability in vitamin K content and hidden food interactions. The primary goal is not to avoid all vitamin K but to keep your intake consistent and avoid large, unanticipated spikes or drops. Familiarize yourself with a "vitamin K scoring" mindset to assess menu choices quickly:

- ***High-Vitamin K Red Flag***: Dishes featuring dark leafy greens such as kale, spinach, collard greens, Swiss chard, or broccoli deserve a "high" score, signaling the need for portion control or substitution.
- ***Moderate-Vitamin K Yellow Zone***: Menu items with peas, asparagus, Brussels sprouts, green beans, or pre-mixed salads containing small amounts of kale or spinach should be considered "moderate." If these foods are frequently part of your weekly meals, small servings can usually fit without issue—but avoid double portions or unexpected extra sides.
- ***Low-Vitamin K Green Light***: Plain proteins (grilled chicken, fish, lean meats, eggs), non-green vegetables (peppers, carrots, mushrooms, squash), grains, potatoes, and fruits are low in vitamin K, making them the safest default options on most menus.

Some practical ordering cues:

- Watch for hidden greens in sandwiches, smoothies, wraps, or grain bowls, which can significantly increase vitamin K content.
- Ask for sauces, dressings, or salads "on the side" so you're in control of portions.
- Check if restaurants can swap out high-vitamin K vegetables for lower alternatives.
- Limit portions of unfamiliar green side dishes if your weekly vitamin K pattern is usually low or moderate.

Checklist for Traveling: Portable Meal and Snack Strategies, Supplement Management

Travel inherently disrupts eating schedules and access to familiar meals, introducing instability in vitamin K and increasing supplement confusion. Use the following checklist to structure your travel preparations:

1. **Plan Ahead:**
    - Pack individual portions of reliable low-vitamin K snacks, such as unsalted nuts, whole-grain crackers, fruit, or prepared snack bars made without hidden greens.
    - Pre-slice carrots, cucumber, apple, or bell pepper sticks in resealable bags for on-the-go snacks.
    - For longer trips, consider preparing a small meal kit with hard-boiled eggs, cooked chicken breast, or whole fruit for the first day, minimizing surprise ingredients.
2. **Supplement Management:**
    - Carry all prescribed supplements and medications in their original labeled containers to avoid confusion during security checks and time changes.
    - Bring an up-to-date list of all supplements, over-the-counter remedies, and herbal products you take, highlighting any with potential

anticoagulant interactions (such as high-dose garlic or turmeric supplements).

- If you routinely take a multivitamin, confirm with your pharmacist that it is appropriate for blood thinner users, as some formulas contain high doses of vitamin K.

3. **Practical Tips:**
   - Always bring a written summary of your dietary needs—in case you need medical attention or restaurant substitutions during your travels.
   - Scout ahead for supermarkets or restaurants near your accommodation that offer "build-your-own" meals, where you can select individual vitamin K–safe ingredients.
   - Consider using a travel cooler or insulated bag if you need to keep certain safe foods fresh during air or road travel.

Meal Customization Template for Social Events or Gatherings with Unknown Foods

When attending gatherings, parties, or any event with unfamiliar or buffet-style food options, a customization approach can protect INR stability without sacrificing social engagement. Here's a simple but effective meal customization template:

- ***Visual Survey***: Upon arrival, take a visual inventory of available foods. Identify dishes high in visible green vegetables or those with unidentifiable blended greens (think dips, pestos, or soups with a green tint).
- ***Smart Plate Building***: Start by serving yourself small portions of low-vitamin K staples proteins, grains, non-green veggies, and fruits then, if desired, add moderate-vitamin K items in the ratios that reflect your at-home habits.
- ***Portion Awareness***: When in doubt about the vitamin K content of a dish (such as a casserole or stew), opt for a smaller serving. If you sample several unknowns, keep the total quantity moderate and avoid double-serving any single green-heavy option.
- ***Logging and Adjustment***: Jot down (in your meal tracker or smartphone) an approximate list of what you ate and any "high or moderate" vitamin K foods consumed. This provides both awareness and a reference point if you need to communicate dietary details to your care team after the event.

Restaurant Conversation Script for Communicating Dietary Needs Without Awkwardness

Advocating for your dietary needs in a restaurant doesn't have to be uncomfortable. A well-prepared script can effectively communicate your requirements while encouraging cooperation from dining staff. Example script:

"I take a medication for my heart rhythm that requires my vitamin K (from greens and some vegetables) to stay about the same most days. Could you let me know if this dish contains spinach, kale, or other dark green vegetables? If so, could I have it made with a different vegetable like carrots, bell peppers, mushrooms, or tomatoes instead?"

Or, for sauces and dressings:

"Since I need to manage my vitamin K intake, could I have any pesto, green sauces, or salad dressings on the side? And could you tell me if there are any unexpected greens blended into the soups or mixed dishes?"

Tips for confident communication:

- Reference your heart medication as the reason for your request, which usually produces understanding rather than skepticism.
- Be polite, brief, and clear. Use specific vegetable names instead of saying "greens," which could be interpreted too loosely.
- Thank the staff for checking with the kitchen and confirming before your meal arrives if your request was understood.

This proactive approach allows you to maintain safety seamlessly and sets the stage for positive, helpful interactions on future visits.

Holiday Meal Planning Worksheet for Managing Buffet-Style or Multi-Course Occasions

Holidays often bring multi-course meals, buffets, or "potluck" tables laden with unpredictable, high-variation foods. Use this worksheet to approach festive eating with confidence and stability:

1. **Pre-Event Planning:**
   - If possible, find out which dishes will be served and whether any contain significant amounts of dark leafy greens or herbs.
   - Volunteer to bring a safe, satisfying low–vitamin K dish that can serve as your "anchor" during the meal (like a vegetable and grain salad without greens, roasted root vegetables, or citrus fruit platters).
2. **At the Event:**
   - Use your vitamin K scoring cues to categorize available foods as "high," "moderate," or "low."
   - Start with the "low" category on your plate: plain proteins, potatoes, grains, and non-green

vegetables. Add moderate items in measured portions if desired.

- Limit total high-vitamin K selections to quantities you would typically eat at home to keep daily variation minimal. If you do opt for a traditional high-vitamin K holiday dish, skip other green foods that day to balance your intake.
- Watch for cumulative effects: Don't double "moderate" servings, thinking one dish alone "won't hurt," as total intake over the meal matters most.

3. **Post-Event Adjustment:**
   - Record which foods and serving sizes you consumed, especially any out-of-the-ordinary vitamin K sources.
   - Be especially attentive to your INR (if on warfarin) for the week following a holiday, as holiday meals can have delayed effects.
   - If you notice instability or symptoms post-holiday, relay your log and concerns to your healthcare provider early for timely advice.

Social eating, travel, and holiday gatherings need not threaten the stability of your anticoagulant therapy for AFib. With sharpened vitamin K awareness, proactive planning, and open communication, you can enjoy these experiences with both safety and confidence. Keep the guide's ordering strategies, travel checklists, meal customization templates, conversation scripts, and event planning worksheets on hand—or saved on your phone for reference whenever you're away from your normal routine.

Ultimately, the key is to identify and control variables within your reach: knowing how to spot high-vitamin K foods, how to advocate for your dietary needs, and how to record and rebalance intake after variable meals. This approach supports your week-to-week consistency, minimizes food–drug interaction risks, and leaves you free to savor the moments that matter, worry-free.

Conclusion

Finding lasting consistency and safety in your food choices is crucial when managing atrial fibrillation (AFib) with blood thinners. Throughout this guide, you've acquired checklists, planning frameworks, and straightforward weekly systems designed specifically to help you maintain reliable vitamin K intake, avoid unexpected food–drug interactions, and support the efficacy of your anticoagulation therapy. It's not just about understanding science , it's about turning that knowledge into everyday habits you can depend on.

Begin by making use of the actionable tools featured in this guide, such as the weekly vitamin K intake tracker, shopping checklists, and meal planning templates. Embracing these systems at home forms a foundation for stable nutritional routines. Regularly review your pantry with the sorting system outlined, removing items that could jeopardize consistency, and replenishing those that align with your medication needs. Simple, scheduled pantry audits every month can prevent accidental consumption of high-interaction foods or supplements. These practical measures reduce the chances of inadvertent dietary changes and keep you on course.

Investing a few minutes each week in tracking your meals and snacks also helps you spot any creeping variation early. Use the suggested meal and supplement trackers to note what you're eating, especially after events or when your routine changes. Such documentation is invaluable not only for your self-awareness but as a communication tool for care providers. When sharing your detailed food logs and symptom notes during appointments, your healthcare team can more accurately pinpoint problems and suggest tailored adjustments.

Successful blood thinner management for AFib hinges on consistency, but flexibility is also key. If you find yourself eating out, traveling, or attending a social gathering, rely on the frameworks you've practiced: assess menu items for vitamin K, use substitution charts, and communicate dietary needs confidently. These skills, built from the guide's ordering and customization scripts, ensure you can navigate unfamiliar situations with steadiness and without unnecessary anxiety.

Keeping up with regular communication with your care providers further safeguards against complications. Transparent sharing of food logs, coupled with ongoing dialogue about dietary changes or unusual symptoms, arms your medical team with the insights necessary for well-informed advice. Don't wait for problems to escalate if you see significant shifts in your INR or symptoms after dietary changes, connect early and share specifics. This proactive communication is a simple yet powerful defense against costly setbacks.

The cumulative impact of these daily and weekly practices is profound. By methodically applying checklists and frameworks to your kitchen, pantry, grocery trips, and dining out experiences, you dramatically improve the reliability of your INR control and reduce the risk of sudden vitamin K or food–drug interaction spikes. This translates directly into greater safety, confidence, and peace of mind, regardless of where or when you eat.

In summary, managing blood thinners for AFib is not solely about restriction, but about routine, vigilance, and adaptation. The tools and systems offered in this guide provide the backbone for reliable self-management. Return to the checklists and meal planning tools regularly. Make them part of your weekly rhythm. When merged with open communication and regular monitoring, these practices empower you to live actively and eat confidently, all while minimizing the risks that come with anticoagulation therapy.

FAQs

How can I keep my vitamin K intake consistent if I eat out often?

Consistency is key for safe blood thinner use, especially with warfarin, which interacts with vitamin K-rich foods. Eating out can add uncertainty, as most menus don't list vitamin K content and preparation methods vary. However, with some planning, you can keep your intake steady.

Aim to eat similar amounts and types of leafy greens and other vitamin K-rich foods each week, whether at home or dining out. For example, if you typically have a spinach or kale salad a few times a week, try to match this routine when eating out. If you plan to eat more or less than usual, tell your healthcare provider, as large changes can affect your INR. You can also ask for dressings or garnishes on the side to control how much you consume.

Some restaurants post nutrition info online and review these in advance to identify high vitamin K foods. If unsure, opt for lower vitamin K vegetables like romaine or iceberg lettuce, carrots, or green beans. Avoid sudden changes in your intake pattern, as big increases or decreases in leafy greens can destabilize your anticoagulation therapy.

Which foods or drinks have the highest risk of interacting with warfarin?

Warfarin interacts with more foods and drinks than newer blood thinners, so knowing high-risk items is important. The biggest risks are foods high in vitamin K, but other interactions matter too.

High-risk foods and drinks include:

- ***Leafy green vegetables***: Kale, spinach, collard greens, swiss chard, and parsley can reduce warfarin's effectiveness if your intake changes suddenly.
- ***Certain herbs and supplements***: Herbal teas with licorice, alfalfa, or green tea, as well as vitamin K-rich supplements and green powders, may interact with warfarin.
- ***Alcohol***: Large or frequent consumption can increase bleeding risk or alter warfarin metabolism.
- ***Cranberry products***: Cranberry juice and supplements may increase bleeding risk.
- ***Grapefruit***: Grapefruit and its juice may affect warfarin metabolism in some people.

Read labels for hidden vitamin K and avoid starting new supplements or herbal teas without medical advice. If you accidentally eat high-risk foods, let your provider know and watch for unusual bruising, bleeding, or INR changes.

Is it safe to eat green vegetables while taking blood thinners for AFib?

Yes. People on blood thinners, including those with AFib, are encouraged to eat green vegetables. The issue isn't eating greens, but making sure your intake is steady. Green vegetables provide important nutrients and fiber for heart health. If you eat leafy greens regularly, keep doing so and let your provider know—your warfarin dose can be adjusted to fit your usual intake. Sudden increases or decreases can destabilize your INR, so aim for consistency.

For those on DOACs, vitamin K fluctuations matter less, but a balanced diet remains important. Communicate any big changes in your diet to your healthcare team.

How do I adjust my diet if my INR levels become unstable?

If your INR is too high or low, first review your recent food intake and any new supplements or medications. Look for sudden changes in the amount or frequency of vitamin K-rich foods. Return to your previously stable eating pattern and log what you eat and drink for several days and share this with your provider to help identify the cause. Avoid drastic changes, such as suddenly cutting out or binging on green vegetables. Instead, focus on gradual, steady routines and seek tailored advice from your care team. Dose adjustments should only be made by your provider.

What supplements should I avoid when on anticoagulant medications?

Some supplements and herbal products can interact with blood thinners, either strengthening or weakening their effect. Risky supplements include:

- Vitamin K-containing supplements: Multivitamins, green powders, or vitamin K pills can counteract warfarin.
- Fish oil and omega-3 supplements: High doses can increase bleeding risk.
- Herbal supplements: St. John's wort, ginkgo, ginseng, dong quai, and high-dose garlic or ginger may alter blood thinner effectiveness.
- Vitamin E: Large doses may increase bleeding risk.

Even "natural" products may contain ingredients that interact with blood thinners. Always check labels and talk to your healthcare team before starting any new supplement.

Does drinking alcohol affect blood thinner medication for AFib?

Alcohol can impact the safety and effectiveness of blood thinners. For those on warfarin, heavy drinking raises bleeding risk and can lead to unstable INR levels. Light to moderate drinking (such as a single glass of wine or beer) may be less risky, but moderation is crucial. For those on DOACs, alcohol can still increase bleeding risk. Share your alcohol habits with your provider for personalized advice, and report any unusual bruising or bleeding after drinking.

Can I follow a vegetarian or vegan diet safely with blood thinners?

Vegetarian and vegan diets can work with blood thinners if well-planned. These diets often include many vitamin K-rich foods. The key is consistency: keep your intake of leafy greens and other high-vitamin K foods steady from week to week. Track what and how much you eat and share this with your provider to help adjust your medication if needed. Watch for fortified foods or supplements that may contain extra vitamin K. Always discuss major dietary changes or new products with your healthcare team.

References and Helpful Links

References and Helpful Links

Couris, R., Tataronis, G., McCloskey, W. et al.. (2006). Dietary Vitamin K Variability Affects International Normalized Ratio (INR) Coagulation Indices. International Journal for Vitamin and Nutrition Research. https://doi.org/10.1024/0300-9831.76.2.65

SUTTIE, J.. (1990). Warfarin and Vitamin K. Clinical Cardiology. https://doi.org/10.1002/clc.1990.13.s6.16

Voukalis, C., Lip, G., Shantsila, E.. (2016). Drug-drug interactions of non-vitamin K oral anticoagulants. Expert Opinion on Drug Metabolism & Toxicology. https://doi.org/10.1080/17425255.2016.1225037

Talasaz, A., McGonagle, B., HajiQasemi, M. et al.. (2024). Pharmacokinetic and Pharmacodynamic Interactions between Food or Herbal Products and Oral Anticoagulants: Evidence Review, Practical Recommendations, and Knowledge Gaps. Seminars in Thrombosis and Hemostasis. https://doi.org/10.1055/s-0044-1790258

Wu, S., Chen, X., Jin, D. et al.. (2018). Warfarin and vitamin K epoxide reductase: a molecular accounting for observed inhibition. Blood. https://doi.org/10.1182/blood-2018-01-830901

Sadler, R., Shoveller, A., Shandilya, U. et al.. (2024). Beyond the Coagulation Cascade: Vitamin K and Its Multifaceted Impact on Human and Domesticated Animal Health. Current Issues in Molecular Biology. https://doi.org/10.3390/cimb46070418

Hollowell, J., Meier, C., Haefeli, W. et al.. (2005). Drug interactions and risk of acute bleeding leading to hospitalisation or death in patients with chronic atrial fibrillation treated with warfarin. Thrombosis and Haemostasis. https://doi.org/10.1160/th05-03-0166

January, C., Wann, L., Calkins, H. et al.. (2019). 2019 AHA/ACC/HRS Focused Update of the 2014 AHA/ACC/HRS Guideline for the Management of Patients With Atrial Fibrillation. Retrieved from https://doi.org/10.1016/j.jacc.2019.01.011Holbrook, A., Schulman, S., Witt, D. et al.. (2012). Evidence-Based Management of Anticoagulant Therapy. https://doi.org/10.1378/chest.11-2295

www.ingramcontent.com/pod-product-compliance
Lightning Source LLC
LaVergne TN
LVHW020235210926
848481LV00016B/2334